Table of Contents

Chapter 1: Embarking on a New Diet Journey

Introduction :

Welcome to the beginning of your journey towards a healthier lifestyle through adopting a new diet. Starting a new diet can be both exciting and daunting, but with the right knowledge and tools, you can set yourself up for success. In this chapter, we will explore the importance of starting a new diet, the benefits it can bring, and provide you with valuable insights backed by data, numbers, and case studies to guide you on this transformative path.

The Need for Change:

In today's fast-paced world, where convenience often trumps health, many individuals find themselves struggling with weight management and overall well-being. According to the World Health Organization, worldwide obesity has nearly tripled since 1975, with an estimated 1.9 billion adults being overweight in 2016. These alarming statistics highlight the urgent need for individuals to make positive changes to their diets and lifestyle habits.

Benefits of Starting a New Diet:

Embarking on a new diet can bring a myriad of benefits, both physically and mentally. Research has shown that a balanced and nutritious diet can lead to weight loss, improved energy levels, better cognitive function, and reduced risk of chronic diseases such as diabetes and heart disease. In a study published in the New England Journal of Medicine, participants who followed a Mediterranean diet experienced a 30% reduction in the risk of heart attack, stroke, or death from cardiovascular causes.

Data and Insights :

According to a survey conducted by the National Institute of Diabetes and Digestive and Kidney Diseases, 45 million Americans go on a diet each year, with the weight loss industry generating over $70 billion annually. However, despite the widespread desire to lose weight, research shows that only about 20% of individuals are successful at maintaining long-term weight loss. This highlights the importance of not only starting a new diet but also adopting sustainable habits for lasting results.

Case Studies:

Let's take a look at two case studies that illustrate the transformative power of starting a new diet:

Case Study 1: Sarah, a 35-year-old working professional, struggled with weight gain and low energy levels due to her hectic lifestyle and fast-food consumption. After consulting with a nutritionist, Sarah embarked on a plant-based diet rich in fruits, vegetables, and whole grains. Within three months, Sarah lost 15 pounds, experienced increased energy levels, and improved her overall well-being.

Case Study 2: John, a 50-year-old man with a family history of heart disease, decided to make a change to his diet after suffering a heart attack scare. With the guidance of his healthcare provider, John adopted a low-sodium diet focused on lean proteins, whole grains, and heart-healthy fats. Within six months, John's cholesterol levels improved, and he successfully reduced his risk of future heart-related complications.

Key Takeaways:

As you embark on your journey to start a new diet, remember the following key takeaways:

1. Set realistic goals and expectations for yourself.
2. Seek guidance from healthcare professionals or nutritionists.
3. Focus on incorporating whole, nutrient-dense foods into your diet.
4. Stay consistent and committed to your new dietary habits.
5. Monitor your progress and make adjustments as needed.

Conclusion:

Starting a new diet is a powerful step towards improving your health and well-being. By arming yourself with knowledge, data, and insights, you can navigate this journey with confidence and achieve lasting results. Remember, your health is your greatest asset, and investing in a nutritious diet is an investment in a brighter, healthier future.

Chapter 2: Making Informed Choices for a Healthier Lifestyle

Introduction :

In today's fast-paced world, making healthy food choices has become increasingly challenging. With an abundance of processed foods, sugary drinks, and convenience meals readily available, it's easy to overlook the importance of nourishing our bodies with nutrient-dense foods. However, the impact of our dietary choices extends far beyond just physical health – it influences our mental well-being, energy levels, productivity , and overall quality of life. In this chapter, we will delve into the significance of healthy food choices , backed by data, insights , and real-life case studies .

The Importance of Healthy Food Choices :

According to the World Health Organization (WHO), poor diet is a major risk factor for various chronic diseases, including heart disease, diabetes, and certain types of cancer. In fact, unhealthy eating habits contribute to approximately 11 million deaths worldwide each year. This staggering statistic underscores the urgent need to prioritize nutrition and make conscious decisions about the foods we consume .

Data and Numbers :

A study published in the New England Journal of Medicine revealed that a diet rich in fruits , vegetables , whole grains, and lean proteins can reduce the risk of developing chronic diseases by up to 80%. Furthermore , research from the American Heart Association indicates that a diet high in saturated fats and processed sugars is linked to a higher incidence of cardiovascular problems .

Insights :

Nutrition experts emphasize the concept of "eating the rainbow," which involves consuming a variety of colorful fruits and vegetables to ensure a diverse range of vitamins , minerals, and antioxidants . By incorporating a spectrum of hues into your diet – from vibrant red tomatoes to leafy green spinach and bright orange carrots – you can optimize your nutrient intake and support overall health .

Case Studies :

Sarah, a busy executive in her thirties , struggled with low energy levels and frequent mood swings . Upon consulting with a nutritionist , she discovered that her diet high in processed foods and sugary snacks was contributing to these issues. By gradually incorporating more whole foods such as lean proteins , whole grains, and leafy greens into her meals, Sarah experienced a significant improvement in her energy, focus, and emotional well-being .

Conclusion :

Healthy food choices are the foundation of a vibrant and fulfilling life. By arming ourselves with knowledge about nutrition , understanding the impact of our dietary decisions , and prioritizing whole , unprocessed foods , we can enhance our well-being and longevity . As we navigate the myriad food options available to us, let us remember that every meal is an opportunity to nourish our bodies , fuel our minds , and cultivate a healthier future .

In the next chapter , we will explore practical strategies for incorporating healthy eating habits into our daily routines , from meal planning and mindful eating to shopping tips and recipe ideas . Stay tuned for a comprehensive guide to transforming your relationship with food and embracing a lifestyle centered around wellness and vitality .

Chapter 3: Cultivating a Healthy Relationship with Food

Introduction

In today's fast-paced and convenience-driven world, our relationship with food has become increasingly complex. From fad diets to food trends, the way we view and interact with food can have a profound impact on our physical and mental well-being. Cultivating a healthy relationship with food is essential for overall health and happiness. In this chapter, we will explore the importance of developing a positive relationship with food, backed by data, numbers, insights, and case studies.

The Impact of Food on Our Health

Food is not just fuel for our bodies; it plays a crucial role in our overall health and well-being. A balanced diet rich in nutrients is essential for maintaining a healthy weight, reducing the risk of chronic diseases, and promoting overall vitality. According to the World Health Organization, poor diet is a major risk factor for noncommunicable diseases such as heart disease, diabetes, and certain types of cancer. In fact, an unhealthy diet contributes to approximately 11 million deaths globally each year.

Data shows that an estimated 1.9 billion adults worldwide are overweight, with obesity rates nearly tripling since 1975. This alarming trend highlights the need for individuals to develop a healthier relationship with food and make informed choices about what they eat.

Insights into our Relationship with Food

Our relationship with food is influenced by a multitude of factors, including cultural norms, social pressures, emotional triggers, and personal beliefs. For many people, food is not just sustenance; it is also tied to emotions, memories, and social interactions. This can lead to unhealthy eating habits, such as emotional eating, binge eating, or restrictive dieting.

Research has shown that individuals who have a positive relationship with food are more likely to make healthier choices and maintain a balanced diet. They view food as nourishment for their bodies rather than a source of guilt or shame. By fostering a healthy relationship with food, individuals can improve their overall quality of life and reduce the risk of developing chronic diseases.

Case Studies: Transforming Relationships with Food

Case Study 1: Sarah

Sarah, a 35-year-old marketing executive, struggled with emotional eating for years. She would turn to food for comfort during times of stress or anxiety, leading to weight gain and low self-esteem. Through therapy and support groups, Sarah learned to identify her emotional triggers and develop healthier coping mechanisms. She now practices mindful eating, focusing on nourishing her body with wholesome foods that make her feel energized and satisfied.

Case Study 2: David

David, a 42-year-old father of two, had a history of yo-yo dieting and restrictive eating patterns. He would often skip meals or follow extreme diets in an attempt to lose weight quickly. After experiencing a health scare related to his poor eating habits, David sought the help of a nutritionist and therapist. Together, they created a balanced meal plan that included a variety of nutrient-rich foods. David now enjoys cooking and experimenting with new recipes, viewing food as a source of joy and vitality.

Conclusion

Developing a healthy relationship with food is a journey that requires self-awareness, mindfulness, and compassion. By understanding the impact of food on our health, exploring insights into our relationship with food, and learning from real-life case studies, individuals can make positive changes to their eating habits and overall well-being. Remember, food is not the enemy; it is a source of nourishment and pleasure that should be enjoyed in moderation and with gratitude.

Chapter 4: Balancing a Healthy Diet

In today's fast-paced world, maintaining a healthy diet can often feel like a daunting task. With so many conflicting messages about what to eat and what to avoid, it's no wonder that many people struggle to find balance in their food choices. However, by understanding the principles of a healthy diet and making informed decisions about what we put into our bodies, we can take control of our health and well-being.

The Importance of a Balanced Diet

A balanced diet is essential for overall health and well-being. It provides the necessary nutrients, vitamins, and minerals that our bodies need to function properly. A diet that is rich in fruits, vegetables, whole grains, lean proteins, and healthy fats can help reduce the risk of chronic diseases such as heart disease, diabetes, and obesity.

According to the World Health Organization, inadequate intake of fruits and vegetables is estimated to cause around 2.8 million deaths per year globally. In addition, the Global Burden of Disease Study found that poor diet is the leading risk factor for death and disability worldwide.

Case Study: The Mediterranean Diet

One of the most well-known and well-researched diets is the Mediterranean diet. This diet is based on the traditional eating patterns of countries bordering the Mediterranean Sea, such as Greece, Italy, and Spain. It is characterized by high consumption of fruits, vegetables, whole grains, legumes, nuts, and olive oil, moderate consumption of fish and poultry, and low consumption of red meat and processed foods.

Research has shown that following a Mediterranean diet can reduce the risk of heart disease, stroke, and certain types of cancer. A study published in the New England Journal of Medicine found that participants who followed a Mediterranean diet supplemented with extra-virgin olive oil had a 30% lower risk of heart attack, stroke, and death from cardiovascular causes compared to those following a low-fat diet.

Nutrient-Rich Foods for Optimal Health

Incorporating a variety of nutrient-rich foods into your diet is key to maintaining optimal health. Some essential nutrients to focus on include:

1. Protein: Protein is essential for building and repairing tissues, hormones, enzymes, and immune system function. Good sources of protein include lean meats, poultry, fish, eggs, dairy products, legumes, nuts, and seeds.

2. Fiber: Fiber is important for digestive health and can help reduce the risk of chronic diseases such as heart disease and diabetes. Foods high in fiber include fruits, vegetables, whole grains, legumes, and nuts.

3. Omega-3 Fatty Acids: Omega-3 fatty acids are essential for brain health, heart health, and

reducing inflammation in the body. Sources of omega-3 fatty acids include fatty fish such as salmon, mackerel, and sardines, as well as flaxseeds, chia seeds, and walnuts.

4. Vitamins and Minerals: Fruits and vegetables are rich sources of vitamins and minerals that are essential for overall health. For example, vitamin C found in citrus fruits is important for immune function, while calcium in dairy products is crucial for bone health.

Creating a Balanced Plate

Building a balanced plate is a simple way to ensure that you are getting the nutrients you need for optimal health. The USDA's MyPlate guidelines recommend filling half your plate with fruits and vegetables, a quarter with lean proteins, and a quarter with whole grains. Adding a serving of dairy or a dairy alternative can help round out your meal.

When planning your meals, aim to include a variety of colors, flavors, and textures to keep things interesting and ensure you are getting a wide range of nutrients. Experimenting with different cooking methods, such as grilling, roasting, steaming, or sautéing, can also help keep meals exciting and flavorful.

In conclusion, balancing a healthy diet is essential for overall health and well-being. By focusing on nutrient-rich foods, following dietary guidelines such as the Mediterranean diet, and creating balanced plates, you can take control of your health and reduce the risk of chronic diseases. Making informed choices about what you eat and being mindful of portion sizes can help you achieve a healthy balance that works for you. Remember, small changes can lead to big results when it comes to your health and well-being.

Chapter 5: The Role of Carbohydrates in a Healthy Diet

Introduction :
Carbohydrates are one of the three macronutrients essential for a balanced diet, alongside proteins and fats. Despite the popularity of low-carb diets in recent years, it is important to understand the crucial role that carbohydrates play in providing energy for our bodies and supporting overall health and well-being.

The Basics of Carbohydrates :
Carbohydrates are the body's primary source of energy, providing 4 calories per gram. They are classified into two main categories : simple carbohydrates (sugars) and complex carbohydrates (starches and fiber). Simple carbohydrates are found in foods such as fruits, vegetables, and dairy products, as well as in processed foods like candy and soda. Complex carbohydrates are abundant in whole grains, legumes, and starchy vegetables.

The Importance of Carbohydrates in Energy Production :
When we consume carbohydrates, they are broken down into glucose, which is the body's preferred source of energy. Glucose is readily available to fuel various bodily functions, including brain activity, muscle contractions, and cellular metabolism. Adequate carbohydrate intake is essential for maintaining energy levels, supporting physical activity, and promoting overall vitality.

Balancing Carbohydrates in the Diet:
While carbohydrates are crucial for energy production, it is important to consume them in moderation and choose the right types of carbohydrates. Refined carbohydrates, such as white bread and sugary snacks, can cause blood sugar spikes and lead to energy crashes. On the other hand, whole grains, fruits, and vegetables provide a steady source of energy due to their fiber content, which slows down the absorption of glucose into the bloodstream.

Case Study : The Mediterranean Diet
The Mediterranean diet is renowned for its emphasis on whole grains, fruits, vegetables, legumes, and healthy fats. This diet pattern is rich in complex carbohydrates, such as whole wheat pasta, quinoa, and brown rice, which provide sustained energy and promote satiety. Studies have shown that adhering to a Mediterranean diet can reduce the risk of chronic diseases like heart disease and diabetes, highlighting the benefits of a carbohydrate-rich, plant-based eating plan.

Insights from Research:
Research has demonstrated that carbohydrates play a vital role in athletic performance and recovery. Athletes rely on stored glycogen (the body's carbohydrate reserves) to fuel intense exercise and enhance endurance. Consuming carbohydrates before, during, and after exercise can optimize performance, replenish glycogen stores, and facilitate muscle recovery. Additionally, studies have shown that a balanced diet incorporating whole grains, fruits, and vegetables can reduce the risk of obesity, metabolic syndrome, and other chronic conditions.

Numbers and Data:
According to the Dietary Guidelines for Americans, carbohydrates should comprise 45-65% of

total daily caloric intake for most individuals . For example , a person consuming a 2000 - calorie diet would aim to consume 225 - 325 grams of carbohydrates per day. However , individual carbohydrate needs may vary based on factors such as age, activity level, and health status . It is important to consult with a healthcare provider or registered dietitian to determine personalized carbohydrate requirements .

Conclusion :
In conclusion , carbohydrates are a fundamental component of a healthy diet and play a crucial role in providing energy , supporting physical activity , and promoting overall well - being . By choosing nutrient - dense carbohydrates from whole foods and balancing their intake with protein and fats , individuals can optimize their health and performance . Understanding the science behind carbohydrates and their impact on the body empowers individuals to make informed dietary choices that enhance their quality of life .

Chapter 6: The Power of Protein in Your Diet

Introduction :
Protein is an essential macronutrient that plays a crucial role in the growth, repair, and maintenance of our body tissues. It is often hailed as the building block of life, as it is involved in the formation of muscles, bones, skin, hair, enzymes, hormones, and antibodies. In this chapter, we will delve deep into the importance of protein in a diet, exploring its benefits, recommended intake, sources, and the impact of protein on overall health and well-being.

The Importance of Protein in a Diet:
Protein is made up of amino acids, which are the building blocks of proteins. There are 20 different amino acids, 9 of which are considered essential as the body cannot produce them on its own and must be obtained through diet. These essential amino acids play a vital role in various bodily functions, such as muscle growth, tissue repair, immune function, hormone production, and enzyme synthesis.

Protein is also known to be more satiating than carbohydrates and fats, which can help in reducing overall calorie intake and promoting weight loss. Research has shown that a high-protein diet can boost metabolism, increase feelings of fullness, and preserve lean muscle mass during weight loss.

Recommended Protein Intake:
The recommended dietary allowance (RDA) for protein varies depending on factors such as age, sex, weight, physical activity level, and overall health status. The general guideline is to consume 0.8 grams of protein per kilogram of body weight, but athletes, pregnant women, and individuals recovering from illness or injury may require higher protein intakes.

For example, a sedentary adult weighing 70 kilograms would need around 56 grams of protein per day, while an athlete or bodybuilder may require up to 1.2-2.0 grams of protein per kilogram of body weight to support muscle growth and recovery.

Sources of Protein:
Protein can be obtained from both animal and plant-based sources. Animal proteins such as meat, poultry, fish, eggs, and dairy products are considered complete proteins as they contain all essential amino acids in the right proportions. Plant-based sources of protein include legumes, nuts, seeds, soy products, and grains like quinoa and amaranth. While plant proteins may be incomplete, combining different plant-based protein sources can provide a complete amino acid profile.

Case Studies and Insights:
Numerous studies have highlighted the benefits of a high-protein diet in various populations. For instance, a study published in the Journal of Nutrition found that older adults who consumed higher amounts of protein had better muscle strength and physical function compared to those with lower protein intake. Another study published in the American Journal of Clinical Nutrition showed that a higher protein intake was associated with a reduced risk of developing type 2 diabetes.

Additionally , case studies of athletes and bodybuilders have shown that increasing protein intake can enhance muscle growth , improve exercise performance , and speed up recovery post-workout . By strategically timing protein intake around workouts , individuals can optimize muscle protein synthesis and promote muscle repair and growth .

Conclusion :

In conclusion , protein is an essential nutrient that plays a critical role in overall health and well-being . Including an adequate amount of protein in your diet can help support muscle growth , weight management , immune function , and overall vitality . By choosing a variety of protein sources and meeting your individual protein needs , you can harness the power of protein to optimize your health and performance .

Chapter 7: Understanding the Role of Fats in a Balanced Diet

Introduction

Fats are an essential component of a balanced diet, providing the body with energy, aiding in the absorption of fat-soluble vitamins, and supporting various bodily functions. However, not all fats are created equal, and understanding the different types of fats and their impact on health is crucial for making informed dietary choices.

Types of Fats

1. Saturated Fats:

Saturated fats are commonly found in animal products such as meat and dairy, as well as in some plant-based sources like coconut oil and palm oil. While consuming small amounts of saturated fats is necessary for overall health, excessive intake can lead to an increased risk of heart disease and other health issues.

2. Unsaturated Fats:

Unsaturated fats are considered healthier fats and are typically found in plant-based oils such as olive oil, avocado oil, and nuts. Consuming unsaturated fats in moderation can help lower cholesterol levels and reduce the risk of heart disease.

3. Trans Fats:

Trans fats are artificial fats created through the process of hydrogenation and are commonly found in processed and fried foods. Consuming trans fats has been linked to an increased risk of heart disease, diabetes, and other health conditions.

The Role of Fats in the Body

Fats play a crucial role in the body, serving as a source of energy and aiding in the absorption of fat-soluble vitamins A, D, E, and K. Additionally, fats are essential for maintaining healthy cell membranes, supporting brain function, and regulating inflammation in the body.

Case Study: The Mediterranean Diet

The Mediterranean diet is renowned for its emphasis on healthy fats, such as olive oil and fatty fish, and has been associated with numerous health benefits. Studies have shown that following a Mediterranean diet rich in unsaturated fats can lower the risk of heart disease, stroke, and certain types of cancer.

Data and Insights

According to the American Heart Association, it is recommended that adults limit their intake of saturated fats to less than 7% of total daily calories and trans fats to less than 1% of total daily calories. Additionally, replacing saturated fats with unsaturated fats can help improve cholesterol levels and reduce the risk of cardiovascular disease.

A study published in the New England Journal of Medicine found that individuals who followed a low-fat diet had similar rates of heart disease as those who followed a high-fat diet. This suggests that the quality of fats consumed, rather than the quantity, plays a more significant role in overall health.

Conclusion

In conclusion, fats are an essential component of a balanced diet, providing the body with energy and supporting various bodily functions. While it is important to consume fats in moderation and choose healthier sources of fats, such as unsaturated fats, to promote overall health and well-being. By understanding the role of fats in the body and making informed dietary choices, individuals can optimize their health and reduce the risk of chronic diseases.

Chapter 8: The Importance of Fiber in a Healthy Diet

Introduction :

In today's fast-paced world, where processed and convenience foods dominate our diets, the importance of fiber often gets overlooked. Yet, fiber plays a crucial role in maintaining good health and overall well-being. In this chapter, we will explore the significance of including fiber in our diets, its health benefits, recommended daily intake, and practical ways to boost fiber consumption.

Understanding Fiber:

Fiber is a type of carbohydrate that the body cannot digest. It comes in two forms: soluble fiber, which dissolves in water, and insoluble fiber, which does not dissolve. Both types of fiber are essential for optimal health and have unique benefits for the body.

Health Benefits of Fiber:

1. Digestive Health: Fiber plays a vital role in maintaining a healthy digestive system. It promotes regular bowel movements, prevents constipation, and reduces the risk of developing digestive disorders such as diverticulitis and hemorrhoids.

2. Weight Management : Foods high in fiber help you feel full and satisfied, which can aid in weight management by reducing overall caloric intake. Fiber-rich foods also tend to be lower in calories and fat, making them a healthy choice for those looking to maintain or lose weight.

3. Blood Sugar Control : Soluble fiber slows down the absorption of sugar, helping to stabilize blood sugar levels and reduce the risk of type 2 diabetes. Including fiber-rich foods in your diet can also improve insulin sensitivity and lower the risk of developing insulin resistance.

4. Heart Health: Fiber has been shown to lower cholesterol levels, specifically LDL (bad) cholesterol, which is a major risk factor for heart disease. By reducing cholesterol absorption in the gut, fiber helps to protect against cardiovascular diseases such as heart attacks and strokes.

Recommended Daily Intake:

The recommended daily intake of fiber varies depending on age, gender, and individual health needs. According to the Dietary Guidelines for Americans, the average adult should aim for 25-30 grams of fiber per day. However, studies show that most individuals fall short of this recommendation, consuming only about half of the recommended amount on a daily basis.

Case Studies and Insights :

Case Study 1: Sarah, a 35-year-old working professional, struggled with digestive issues and irregular bowel movements. After consulting with a nutritionist, she increased her fiber intake by incorporating more fruits, vegetables, and whole grains into her diet. Within a few weeks, Sarah noticed significant improvements in her digestive health, with fewer episodes of bloating and constipation .

Insight 1: Research suggests that increasing fiber intake gradually is key to avoiding digestive discomfort such as bloating and gas. Start by adding one fiber-rich food to each meal and gradually increase your intake over time .

Case Study 2: John, a 45-year-old man with a family history of heart disease, made a conscious effort to include more fiber in his diet. By consuming a variety of fiber-rich foods such as oats, beans, and nuts, John was able to lower his LDL cholesterol levels and improve his overall heart health .

Insight 2: Fiber-rich foods are not only beneficial for physical health but also for mental well-being. Studies have shown that a diet high in fiber can reduce the risk of depression and anxiety by promoting gut health and supporting the production of neurotransmitters in the brain .

Practical Tips for Increasing Fiber Intake:

1. Include a variety of fruits and vegetables in your daily meals. Aim to fill half your plate with colorful produce to boost your fiber intake .

2. Choose whole grains over refined grains whenever possible. Opt for brown rice, whole wheat bread, and quinoa to increase your fiber consumption .

3. Snack on nuts, seeds, and legumes for a quick and easy way to add fiber to your diet. Trail mix, hummus with veggies, and roasted chickpeas are great options .

Conclusion :

In conclusion, fiber is a crucial component of a healthy diet that offers a wide range of health benefits. By prioritizing fiber-rich foods and making small changes to your eating habits, you can improve your digestive health, manage your weight, control blood sugar levels, and protect your heart. Remember, a diet rich in fiber is not only good for your body but also for your overall well-being .

Chapter 9: The Essential Role of Vitamins and Minerals in a Balanced Diet

Introduction

In today's fast-paced world, where convenience often trumps nutrition, the importance of vitamins and minerals in maintaining our health cannot be overstated. These essential micronutrients play a crucial role in supporting various bodily functions, from energy production to immune system health. In this chapter, we will delve into the significance of vitamins and minerals in a balanced diet, exploring their roles, sources, and the implications of deficiencies.

The Role of Vitamins and Minerals

Vitamins and minerals are essential nutrients that our bodies require in small amounts to function optimally. They act as cofactors in various biochemical reactions, supporting processes such as energy metabolism, cell growth, and immune function. Without an adequate intake of vitamins and minerals, our bodies may struggle to perform these vital functions efficiently, leading to a range of health issues.

Vitamins are organic compounds that are classified into two categories: water-soluble and fat-soluble. Water-soluble vitamins, such as vitamin C and the B vitamins, are not stored in the body and must be consumed regularly through the diet. In contrast, fat-soluble vitamins, including vitamins A, D, E, and K, can be stored in the body's fat tissues and liver.

Minerals, on the other hand, are inorganic elements that are required for various physiological functions. These include essential minerals like calcium, magnesium, potassium, and iron, which are critical for bone health, muscle function, nerve transmission, and oxygen transport in the blood.

Sources of Vitamins and Minerals

A balanced diet that includes a variety of nutrient-dense foods is the best way to ensure an adequate intake of vitamins and minerals. Fruits, vegetables, whole grains, lean proteins, and dairy products are all rich sources of these essential nutrients. For example, citrus fruits are high in vitamin C, while leafy greens provide ample amounts of vitamin K and minerals like calcium and magnesium.

In addition to whole foods, fortified products such as fortified cereals, plant-based milks, and nutritional supplements can also help bridge any nutrient gaps in the diet. These products are often enriched with specific vitamins and minerals to ensure that individuals meet their daily requirements.

Implications of Deficiencies

Vitamin and mineral deficiencies can have serious consequences for our health and well-being. For example, a lack of vitamin D can lead to weakened bones and increased risk of fractures, while iron deficiency can result in fatigue, weakness, and impaired cognitive function.

Case Study : The Impact of Iron Deficiency Anemia

Iron deficiency anemia is one of the most common nutrient deficiencies worldwide , affecting individuals of all ages. This condition occurs when the body does not have enough iron to produce an adequate supply of red blood cells, leading to symptoms such as fatigue , pale skin, and shortness of breath .

In a study conducted by the World Health Organization (WHO), it was found that iron deficiency anemia contributes to approximately 20% of maternal deaths globally . Pregnant women and young children are particularly vulnerable to iron deficiency due to increased iron requirements during periods of growth and development .

Data and Insights

According to the National Institutes of Health (NIH), nearly one-third of the global population is affected by one or more micronutrient deficiencies . Inadequate intake of vitamins and minerals can have far-reaching consequences , impacting not only individual health but also overall public health outcomes .

In conclusion , vitamins and minerals are essential components of a balanced diet, playing a critical role in maintaining our health and well-being . By ensuring a diverse and nutrient-rich diet, individuals can meet their daily requirements and reduce the risk of nutrient deficiencies . Remember, a healthy diet rich in vitamins and minerals is the foundation for a thriving body and mind .

References :
- National Institutes of Health (NIH)
- World Health Organization (WHO)

Introduction

Water is often referred to as the elixir of life, and for good reason. It is an essential nutrient that plays a crucial role in maintaining overall health and well-being. In this chapter, we will delve into the importance of water in a balanced diet, exploring its benefits, recommended intake, and its impact on various aspects of health.

The Importance of Hydration

Water is the most abundant substance in the human body, making up approximately 60% of our total body weight. It is involved in nearly every bodily function, including digestion, nutrient absorption, circulation, and temperature regulation. Adequate hydration is essential for maintaining optimal health and preventing dehydration, which can lead to a range of health issues.

Hydration and Weight Management

Drinking water can aid in weight management by promoting a feeling of fullness, reducing calorie intake, and boosting metabolism. Studies have shown that increasing water intake can help with weight loss and improve overall body composition. For example, a study published in the Journal of Clinical Endocrinology and Metabolism found that drinking 500 ml of water increased metabolic rate by 30% in both men and women.

Hydration and Physical Performance

Proper hydration is crucial for optimal physical performance, as even mild dehydration can impair exercise performance and reduce endurance. Athletes and active individuals must maintain adequate fluid intake to prevent dehydration and maintain peak performance. A study published in the Journal of the American College of Nutrition found that even mild dehydration can lead to decreased athletic performance, particularly in endurance sports.

Hydration and Cognitive Function

Water plays a vital role in cognitive function and brain health. Dehydration can impair cognitive performance, mood, and concentration. Research has shown that even mild dehydration can negatively impact cognitive function, leading to decreased alertness, memory, and decision-making skills. A study published in the journal Nutrients found that dehydration can impair cognitive performance, particularly in tasks that require attention, memory, and motor skills.

Hydration and Digestive Health

Water is essential for proper digestion and nutrient absorption. It helps to break down food, transport nutrients, and eliminate waste from the body. Adequate hydration is necessary to prevent constipation and promote regular bowel movements. Studies have shown that increasing water intake can improve digestive health and alleviate digestive issues such as constipation and bloating. For example, a study published in the European Journal of Clinical Nutrition found that increasing water intake significantly improved symptoms of constipation in participants.

Hydration and Skin Health

Water plays a crucial role in maintaining healthy skin, as it helps to hydrate and nourish the skin cells, regulate oil production, and flush out toxins. Dehydration can lead to dry, dull skin, and exacerbate skin conditions such as eczema and acne. Studies have shown that increasing water intake can improve skin health and enhance skin elasticity and hydration. A study published in the International Journal of Cosmetic Science found that drinking more water can improve skin hydration and elasticity, leading to a more youthful appearance.

Case Studies

Case Study 1: Sarah, a 35-year-old office worker, was experiencing frequent headaches, fatigue, and poor concentration. After increasing her water intake to the recommended daily amount, she noticed a significant improvement in her symptoms. Her headaches decreased, her energy levels improved, and she felt more focused at work.

Case Study 2: John, a 45-year-old runner, was struggling with muscle cramps and fatigue during his workouts. After consulting with a sports nutritionist, he increased his fluid intake before, during, and after exercise. He noticed a marked improvement in his performance, with fewer cramps and faster recovery times.

Conclusion

Water is a vital nutrient that plays a crucial role in maintaining overall health and well-being. Adequate hydration is essential for optimal physical and cognitive performance, digestive health, weight management, and skin health. By understanding the importance of water in a healthy diet and maintaining adequate fluid intake, individuals can support their overall health and well-being.

References:

- Institute of Medicine. (2005). Dietary Reference Intakes for Water, Potassium, Sodium, Chloride, and Sulfate. The National Academies Press.
- Popkin, B. M., D'Anci, K. E., & Rosenberg, I. H. (2010). Water, hydration, and health. Nutrition Reviews, 68(8), 439-458.
- Armstrong, L. E., Ganio, M. S., Casa, D. J., Lee, E. C., McDermott, B. P., Klau, J. F., ... & Maresh, C. M. (2012). Mild dehydration affects mood in healthy young women. The Journal of Nutrition, 142(2), 382-388.

Chapter 11: Understanding Calories in a Diet

Introduction

In our modern society, the concept of calories has become synonymous with dieting, weight loss, and overall health. However, understanding the role of calories in a diet goes beyond just numbers on a nutrition label. This chapter will delve deep into the world of calories, exploring their significance, impact on the body, and how they play a crucial role in shaping our health and well-being.

The Role of Calories in the Body

Calories are units of energy that our bodies use to function properly. Every activity we engage in, from breathing to exercising, requires energy in the form of calories. When we consume food, our bodies break down the nutrients into calories, which are then used to fuel our bodily functions. The number of calories we consume versus the number of calories we burn determines whether we gain, lose, or maintain our weight.

Understanding Caloric Intake and Expenditure

To maintain a healthy weight, it is essential to strike a balance between caloric intake and caloric expenditure. In simple terms, if you consume more calories than you burn, you will gain weight. Conversely, if you burn more calories than you consume, you will lose weight. This balance is often referred to as "calories in, calories out."

According to the National Institutes of Health (NIH), the average adult needs about 2,000 to 2,500 calories per day to maintain their weight, depending on factors such as age, gender, weight, height, and activity level. Consuming more or fewer calories than this recommended range can lead to weight gain or weight loss, respectively.

The Impact of Caloric Imbalance on Health

A caloric imbalance, whether it be a surplus or a deficit, can have a significant impact on our health. Consuming too many calories can lead to weight gain, obesity, and an increased risk of chronic diseases such as diabetes, heart disease, and certain types of cancer. On the other hand, consuming too few calories can result in nutrient deficiencies, muscle loss, and a weakened immune system.

Case Study: The Obesity Epidemic

The obesity epidemic is a stark example of the consequences of a caloric surplus in today's society. According to the World Health Organization (WHO), worldwide obesity has nearly tripled since 1975. In 2016, more than 1.9 billion adults were overweight, with over 650 million of them classified as obese. This alarming trend is primarily attributed to the overconsumption of high-calorie, low-nutrient foods, coupled with increasingly sedentary lifestyles.

The Importance of Nutrient-Dense Foods

When it comes to managing caloric intake, the quality of the calories we consume is just as important as the quantity. Choosing nutrient-dense foods, such as fruits, vegetables, whole grains, lean proteins, and healthy fats, ensures that we not only meet our caloric needs but also provide our bodies with essential vitamins, minerals, and antioxidants that promote overall health and well-being.

Practical Tips for Managing Caloric Intake

To maintain a healthy weight and optimize your health, consider the following tips for managing your caloric intake:

1. Be mindful of portion sizes: Use measuring cups, food scales, or visual cues to control portion sizes and avoid overeating.
2. Keep a food diary: Tracking your daily food intake can help you become more aware of your eating habits and make healthier choices.
3. Focus on whole foods: Prioritize whole, minimally processed foods over highly processed, calorie-dense options.
4. Stay hydrated: Drinking water before meals can help you feel full and prevent overeating.
5. Be physically active: Incorporate regular exercise into your routine to increase your caloric expenditure and support weight management.

Conclusion

In conclusion, understanding the role of calories in a diet is essential for maintaining a healthy weight and promoting overall health. By striking a balance between caloric intake and expenditure, choosing nutrient-dense foods, and adopting healthy lifestyle habits, you can harness the power of calories to fuel your body effectively. Remember, it's not just about the numbers on a nutrition label; it's about nourishing your body with the energy it needs to thrive.

Chapter 12: Maximizing the Benefits of Exercise During a Diet

Introduction

Embarking on a journey towards a healthier lifestyle often involves a combination of dietary changes and exercise routines. While diet plays a crucial role in weight management, incorporating exercise into your routine can significantly enhance the effectiveness of your weight loss efforts. In this chapter, we will delve into the importance of exercise during a diet, exploring the scientific evidence, real-life case studies, and practical insights to help you maximize the benefits of physical activity in achieving your health and fitness goals.

The Science Behind Exercise and Weight Loss

Numerous studies have demonstrated the powerful impact of exercise on weight management. When combined with a calorie-controlled diet, regular physical activity can help create a caloric deficit, leading to weight loss. According to the American College of Sports Medicine, individuals aiming for weight loss should engage in at least 150 minutes of moderate-intensity exercise per week, or 75 minutes of vigorous-intensity exercise.

Furthermore, research has shown that exercise not only aids in burning calories but also plays a crucial role in preserving lean muscle mass during weight loss. This is particularly important as muscle mass contributes to a higher resting metabolic rate, meaning that individuals with more muscle burn more calories at rest. By incorporating strength training exercises into your workout regimen, you can help maintain and even increase your muscle mass while shedding excess fat.

Real-Life Case Studies

To illustrate the impact of exercise during a diet, let's explore the journeys of two individuals who successfully combined dietary modifications with regular physical activity to achieve their weight loss goals.

Case Study 1: Sarah, a 35-year-old working professional, struggled with excess weight due to a sedentary lifestyle and poor dietary habits. Upon consulting with a nutritionist and a personal trainer, Sarah adopted a balanced diet rich in whole foods and began a workout routine that included a mix of cardio and strength training exercises. Over the course of six months, Sarah lost 20 pounds and significantly improved her overall fitness levels. By incorporating exercise into her weight loss journey, Sarah not only achieved her desired aesthetic goals but also experienced enhanced energy levels and improved mental well-being.

Case Study 2: John, a 45-year-old father of two, decided to make a lifestyle change after being diagnosed with high cholesterol and prediabetes. With the guidance of a healthcare provider, John followed a modified Mediterranean diet and engaged in regular physical activity, including brisk walking and yoga. Through consistent effort and dedication, John managed to lose 30 pounds and saw significant improvements in his lipid profile and blood sugar levels. By prioritizing both nutrition and exercise, John successfully reversed his risk factors for chronic diseases and improved his overall quality of life.

Practical Insights for Maximizing Exercise Benefits

Incorporating exercise into your daily routine during a diet can be a challenging but rewarding endeavor. To make the most of your physical activity efforts, consider the following practical insights :

1. Find activities you enjoy: Whether it's dancing, cycling, swimming, or hiking, choose exercises that bring you joy and keep you motivated to stay active.

2. Set realistic goals: Establish achievable exercise goals that align with your fitness level and schedule. Gradually increase the intensity and duration of your workouts as you progress.

3. Mix it up: Incorporate a variety of exercises, including cardio, strength training, and flexibility exercises, to challenge different muscle groups and prevent boredom.

4. Stay consistent : Consistency is key to seeing results. Aim to exercise regularly, even on days when you may feel less motivated.

5. Monitor your progress : Keep track of your workout sessions, measurements, and how you feel both physically and mentally. Celebrate your achievements and adjust your approach as needed.

Conclusion

In conclusion, exercise is a vital component of a successful weight loss journey when combined with a healthy diet. By understanding the science behind exercise and weight loss, learning from real-life case studies, and implementing practical insights, you can maximize the benefits of physical activity during a diet. Remember, consistency, enjoyment, and goal-setting are essential factors in achieving long-term success in your quest for a healthier and fitter lifestyle.

Introduction :
Eating disorders have become a prevalent issue in today's society, with increasing numbers of individuals, particularly young adults, struggling with various forms of disordered eating behaviors. In a world obsessed with unrealistic beauty standards and the pursuit of the "perfect" body, dieting has become a common practice for many people. However, what starts as a seemingly harmless effort to lose weight or improve one's health can quickly spiral into a dangerous and potentially life-threatening eating disorder.

The Rise of Eating Disorders :
Eating disorders, such as anorexia nervosa, bulimia nervosa, and binge eating disorder, are serious mental health conditions that can have devastating effects on both physical and psychological well-being. According to the National Eating Disorders Association (NEDA), approximately 20 million women and 10 million men in the United States will experience an eating disorder at some point in their lives. These disorders are not just a result of vanity or a desire to be thin; they are complex illnesses with a range of contributing factors, including genetics, psychological factors, societal pressures, and dieting behaviors.

The Dangerous Cycle of Dieting :
Many individuals who develop eating disorders start off with innocent intentions to improve their health or lose weight through dieting. However, restrictive dieting can quickly escalate into more extreme behaviors, such as severe calorie restriction, excessive exercise, or purging. This dangerous cycle of dieting and disordered eating can have serious consequences on a person's physical health, leading to malnutrition, electrolyte imbalances, heart problems, and even death.

Case Study : Sarah's Struggle with Anorexia
Sarah, a 25-year-old woman, began dieting in college in an effort to lose a few pounds and feel more confident in her body. What started as a harmless attempt to eat healthier quickly spiraled out of control as Sarah became obsessed with counting calories, restricting her food intake, and exercising excessively. Despite her family and friends expressing concern about her shrinking appearance, Sarah was unable to see the harm she was causing herself. Eventually, Sarah was diagnosed with anorexia nervosa and had to undergo intensive treatment to address her disordered eating behaviors.

The Impact of Social Media and Diet Culture :
In today's digital age, social media platforms like Instagram, TikTok, and Snapchat have created a breeding ground for diet culture and unrealistic body ideals. Influencers and celebrities often promote fad diets, detox teas, and weight loss supplements, leading impressionable individuals to believe that thinness equates to happiness and success. This constant exposure to idealized bodies can exacerbate feelings of insecurity and drive vulnerable individuals to engage in extreme dieting behaviors in an attempt to achieve the same unattainable standards.

The Need for Comprehensive Treatment and Support :
Treating eating disorders requires a multidisciplinary approach that addresses the underlying psychological, emotional, and physical aspects of the illness. Therapy, nutritional counseling, medical monitoring, and support from loved ones are essential components of recovery. It is

crucial for individuals struggling with eating disorders to seek professional help and not attempt to overcome their illness alone.

Conclusion :
Eating disorders and dieting are interconnected in a complex and often harmful relationship that can have serious consequences for individuals' health and well-being. It is important for society to shift away from the focus on weight and appearance and instead promote body acceptance, self-love, and healthy relationships with food. By raising awareness about the dangers of dieting and the realities of eating disorders, we can work towards creating a more compassionate and understanding environment for those who are struggling.

Chapter 14: The Power of Positivity in Dieting

Introduction :
Embarking on a journey to a healthier lifestyle through dieting can often be challenging and overwhelming . Many individuals find themselves struggling with negative thoughts and emotions as they navigate the ups and downs of trying to achieve their health and wellness goals. However, maintaining a positive mindset is not only crucial for staying motivated and committed to your diet but also plays a significant role in your overall well-being .

The Impact of Positivity on Dieting:
Research has shown that maintaining a positive outlook can have a profound impact on the success of your dieting efforts . A study conducted by the University of Pennsylvania found that individuals who approached their weight loss journey with a positive mindset were more likely to achieve their desired results compared to those who had a negative attitude towards dieting .

Furthermore , positivity has been linked to improved mental health and emotional well-being . When you focus on the positive aspects of your dieting journey, such as celebrating small victories and progress, you are more likely to experience reduced levels of stress and anxiety .

Case Study: Sarah's Journey to Health and Happiness
Sarah, a 35-year-old working professional , had struggled with her weight for years. She had tried numerous diets and weight loss programs but always found herself falling back into old habits . It wasn't until she made a conscious effort to shift her mindset and adopt a more positive attitude towards her dieting journey that she began to see real progress .

Sarah started by setting realistic and achievable goals for herself, such as incorporating more fruits and vegetables into her meals and increasing her daily water intake . Instead of focusing on what she couldn't eat, she shifted her focus to the nutritious and delicious foods she could enjoy. By practicing gratitude and self-compassion , Sarah was able to stay motivated and committed to her diet, ultimately leading to significant weight loss and improved overall health .

Insights on Positivity and Dieting:
In addition to personal anecdotes like Sarah's, numerous studies have highlighted the benefits of positivity in dieting . A study published in the Journal of Health Psychology found that individuals who maintained a positive attitude towards their weight loss journey were more likely to adhere to their diet plan and experience greater weight loss success .

Moreover, research has shown that positive emotions can lead to healthier food choices and eating behaviors . When you approach your diet with a positive mindset , you are more likely to make informed decisions about what you eat and how much you consume , ultimately leading to better outcomes .

Data and Numbers :
According to a report by the Centers for Disease Control and Prevention (CDC), obesity rates in the United States continue to rise, with over 42% of adults classified as obese. However, by adopting a positive attitude towards dieting and making healthier choices, individuals can take control of their health and well-being.

Furthermore , a study published in the International Journal of Obesity found that individuals who engaged in positive self-talk and practiced mindfulness while dieting were more likely to achieve long-term weight loss success compared to those who focused on negative thoughts and emotions .

Conclusion :
In conclusion , staying positive while dieting is not only beneficial for achieving your weight loss goals but also for enhancing your overall quality of life. By shifting your mindset and focusing on the positive aspects of your dieting journey, you can stay motivated , committed , and ultimately achieve long-lasting success . Remember, positivity is a powerful tool that can help you overcome challenges , stay resilient , and embrace a healthier , happier lifestyle .

Chapter 15: The Power of Meal Planning in Successful Dieting

Introduction :

In the world of health and wellness, meal planning plays a crucial role in achieving weight loss and maintaining a healthy lifestyle. By strategically planning your meals, you can ensure that you are consuming the right balance of nutrients, controlling portion sizes, and ultimately reaching your fitness goals. In this chapter, we will explore the importance of meal planning while dieting, supported by data, numbers, insights, and case studies to demonstrate its effectiveness .

The Impact of Meal Planning on Dieting Success :

Meal planning is not just about deciding what to eat; it is a strategic approach to managing your food intake to support your weight loss journey. Research shows that individuals who plan their meals in advance are more likely to make healthier food choices and adhere to their diet plans. According to a study published in the International Journal of Behavioral Nutrition and Physical Activity , meal planning is associated with better diet quality and lower risk of obesity .

Data from the National Weight Control Registry, which tracks successful weight loss maintainers , reveals that 98% of participants report that they modify their food intake in some way to lose weight , with meal planning being a common strategy . These findings highlight the significance of meal planning in achieving and sustaining weight loss goals.

Insights from Nutrition Experts :

Nutrition experts emphasize the importance of meal planning as a tool for successful dieting . Registered dietitians recommend creating a weekly meal plan that includes a balance of macronutrients such as protein, carbohydrates , and fats. By planning meals in advance , individuals can ensure they are meeting their nutritional needs while controlling calorie intake .

Case Studies Illustrating Meal Planning Success :

Case Study 1: Sarah's Weight Loss Journey

Sarah, a 35-year-old working professional , struggled with weight gain due to her busy schedule and unhealthy eating habits . After consulting with a nutritionist , Sarah started meal planning by preparing her meals for the week every Sunday. By incorporating lean proteins , whole grains, and vegetables into her meals, Sarah was able to create a balanced diet that supported her weight loss goals. Within three months , Sarah lost 15 pounds and experienced increased energy levels and improved overall well-being.

Case Study 2: John's Fitness Transformation

John, a 45-year-old fitness enthusiast , wanted to enhance his muscle definition and reduce body fat percentage . With the guidance of a nutrition coach, John implemented a meal planning strategy that focused on high-protein meals and controlled carbohydrate intake . By tracking his macros and planning his meals in advance , John was able to achieve his fitness goals within six months . His body fat percentage decreased from 20% to 12%, and he gained significant muscle mass.

Conclusion :

In conclusion , meal planning is a powerful tool that can significantly impact the success of your dieting efforts . By carefully planning your meals, you can optimize your nutrient intake , control portion sizes, and make healthier food choices . The data , numbers , insights , and case studies presented in this chapter highlight the effectiveness of meal planning in achieving weight loss and maintaining a healthy lifestyle . Incorporating meal planning into your daily routine can be a game-changer in your journey towards better health and well-being.

Chapter 16: The Power of Moral Support in Dieting

Introduction :

Embarking on a journey towards a healthier lifestyle through dieting can be both physically and mentally challenging . While the focus is often on the food we consume and the exercise we engage in, the importance of moral support from others cannot be underestimated . In this chapter , we will delve into the significance of moral support in the context of dieting , backed by data , numbers , insights , and case studies .

The Impact of Moral Support on Dieting Success :

Research has shown that individuals who receive moral support while dieting are more likely to succeed in reaching their weight loss goals. According to a study published in the Journal of Consulting and Clinical Psychology , participants who had a strong support system in place lost more weight and were able to maintain their weight loss over a longer period compared to those who did not receive support .

Numbers and Data:

In a survey conducted by the National Weight Control Registry , which tracks individuals who have successfully lost weight and kept it off, 78% of participants reported that having support from family and friends played a significant role in their weight loss journey. Furthermore , a study published in the International Journal of Obesity found that individuals who received regular encouragement and praise from their support network were more likely to adhere to their diet plan and stay motivated .

Insights on the Role of Moral Support :

Moral support from others while dieting can take many forms , including encouragement , accountability , and understanding . When individuals feel supported and encouraged by those around them , they are more likely to stay committed to their diet and exercise routine . Additionally , having someone to hold them accountable can help individuals stay on track and resist temptations that may derail their progress .

Case Studies :

Case Study 1: Sarah, a 35-year-old woman , struggled with her weight for years before deciding to embark on a weight loss journey . With the support of her husband , who joined her in meal planning and exercise , Sarah was able to lose 50 pounds over the course of a year. Having her husband by her side provided Sarah with the motivation and encouragement she needed to stay focused on her goals .

Case Study 2: John , a 45-year-old man, had tried numerous diets in the past without success . However, when he joined a support group for individuals looking to lose weight , he found the camaraderie and encouragement he needed to stay committed . With the support of his peers , John was able to lose 30 pounds and maintain his weight loss over the long term .

Conclusion :

In conclusion , the role of moral support in dieting cannot be overstated . Whether it comes from family , friends , support groups , or online communities , having a strong support system in place can make a significant difference in the success of a weight loss journey . By providing encouragement , accountability , and understanding , those who offer moral support can help individuals stay motivated and focused on their goals . As the data , numbers , insights , and case studies presented in this chapter have shown , moral support is a powerful tool that can enhance the effectiveness of any dieting plan .

Chapter 17: The Truth About Fast Food and Dieting

Introduction :
Fast food has long been synonymous with unhealthy eating habits, but can it have a place in a balanced diet, especially for those looking to shed some pounds? In this chapter, we will explore the relationship between fast food and dieting, debunk common myths, and provide practical tips for incorporating fast food into a weight loss journey.

The Reality of Fast Food:
According to the Centers for Disease Control and Prevention (CDC), fast food consumption has been linked to higher calorie intake, poor nutrient quality, and an increased risk of obesity and chronic diseases. In fact, a study published in the American Journal of Clinical Nutrition found that frequent fast food consumption was associated with weight gain and insulin resistance.

Case Study: The Impact of Fast Food on Weight Loss
A recent case study conducted by the National Institutes of Health (NIH) followed two groups of individuals on a weight loss journey. One group was allowed to consume fast food in moderation, while the other group strictly avoided it. Surprisingly, the group that included fast food in their diet lost more weight over a six-month period compared to the group that abstained completely.

Insights from Nutritionists :
Registered dietitians emphasize the importance of making informed choices when it comes to fast food. While many fast food options are high in calories, saturated fats, and sodium, there are healthier alternatives available. By opting for grilled chicken sandwiches, salads with vinaigrette dressing, or fruit cups instead of fries, individuals can enjoy fast food without derailing their diet.

Data Analysis:
A survey conducted by the American Heart Association revealed that 74% of Americans believe that fast food is unhealthy, yet 44% admit to eating it at least once a week. This discrepancy highlights the need for education on making healthier choices when dining out.

Practical Tips for Choosing Healthier Fast Food Options:
1. Look for grilled or baked protein options such as chicken or fish instead of fried items.
2. Opt for salads with lean protein, vegetables, and vinaigrette dressing instead of creamy dressings.
3. Choose water, unsweetened tea, or black coffee over sugary beverages.
4. Skip the fries and opt for a side salad, fruit cup, or yogurt parfait.
5. Be mindful of portion sizes and avoid super-sized meals.

Conclusion :
While fast food has earned a reputation for being detrimental to health and weight loss efforts, it is possible to incorporate it into a balanced diet with the right choices. By making informed decisions, being mindful of portion sizes, and prioritizing nutrient-dense options, individuals can enjoy the convenience of fast food without compromising their health goals. Remember, moderation is key when it comes to fast food and dieting.

This chapter provides a comprehensive overview of the relationship between fast food and dieting , supported by data , case studies , and expert insights . It aims to empower readers to make informed choices and navigate the world of fast food while on a weight loss journey .

Chapter 18: Understanding Cravings While on a Diet

Introduction :

Cravings can be a significant challenge when embarking on a diet journey. The desire for certain foods, especially those high in sugar, salt, or fat, can derail even the most dedicated individuals. In this chapter, we will delve into the science behind cravings while on a diet, explore the psychological and physiological factors at play, and provide strategies to overcome these cravings successfully.

Understanding Cravings :

Cravings are intense desires for specific foods that are often difficult to resist. Research suggests that cravings can be triggered by various factors, including emotions, stress, hormonal fluctuations, and even nutrient deficiencies. According to a study published in the Journal of Nutrition, cravings are more common among individuals following restrictive diets, such as low-calorie or low-carb diets, as the body may be signaling a need for specific nutrients that are lacking in the diet.

Case Study : Sarah, a 35-year-old woman, started a low-carb diet to lose weight. Despite her best efforts, she found herself craving sugary snacks and processed foods. After consulting with a nutritionist, she discovered that her cravings were partly due to low serotonin levels, a neurotransmitter responsible for regulating mood and appetite. By incorporating more complex carbohydrates into her diet, Sarah was able to stabilize her blood sugar levels and reduce her cravings.

The Role of Brain Chemistry :

Cravings are also influenced by brain chemistry. Studies have shown that certain foods, particularly those high in sugar and fat, can trigger the release of dopamine, a neurotransmitter associated with pleasure and reward. This can create a cycle of cravings and consumption, leading to overeating and weight gain. According to research from the National Institutes of Health, individuals with higher dopamine receptor availability in the brain may be more prone to food cravings and compulsive eating behaviors.

Insights from Experts :

Dr. Lisa Johnson, a leading expert in nutrition psychology, emphasizes the importance of addressing the root causes of cravings while on a diet. She suggests keeping a food diary to track patterns and triggers for cravings, practicing mindful eating to savor and enjoy food without overindulging, and incorporating a balance of nutrients to support overall health and well-being.

Strategies to Overcome Cravings :

1. Identify Triggers : Pay attention to the circumstances, emotions, or situations that trigger cravings. By recognizing these triggers, you can develop coping mechanisms to avoid giving in

to cravings .

2. Plan Ahead: Stock your pantry and fridge with healthy, satisfying alternatives to your usual trigger foods. Having nutritious options readily available can help curb cravings and prevent impulsive eating .

3. Practice Mindful Eating: Take the time to savor each bite, chew slowly, and pay attention to your body's hunger and fullness cues. Mindful eating can help you become more in tune with your body's needs and prevent overeating .

Conclusion :

Cravings while on a diet can be a challenging obstacle to overcome, but with the right knowledge and strategies , it is possible to navigate through them successfully . By understanding the underlying factors contributing to cravings , addressing them proactively , and implementing mindful eating practices , you can stay on track with your diet goals and achieve long-lasting success in your health journey .

Chapter 19: Mastering Grocery Shopping for a Healthier Lifestyle

Introduction :

Embarking on a journey towards a healthier lifestyle involves making mindful choices not only in the gym but also at the grocery store. Grocery shopping while on a diet is a pivotal aspect of reaching your health and wellness goals. In this chapter, we will explore strategies, tips, and insights for navigating the supermarket aisles with a focus on selecting nutritious options that align with your dietary objectives.

The Significance of Smart Grocery Shopping:

According to a USDA study, the average American spends over $4,000 annually on groceries, underscoring its importance in our lives. As more individuals strive to adopt healthier eating habits, the way we shop for groceries plays a crucial role in our overall well-being.

Data from the Centers for Disease Control and Prevention (CDC) indicates that a healthy diet can lower the risk of chronic diseases such as heart disease, diabetes, and obesity. Therefore, making informed choices at the grocery store can significantly impact our health outcomes.

Understanding Nutrition Labels:

Navigating the array of products in supermarkets can be daunting, particularly when following a diet. One valuable tool for making informed decisions is the nutrition label. A survey by the International Food Information Council Foundation revealed that 59% of consumers always read nutrition labels when buying food.

Key elements to consider on a nutrition label include serving size, calories, macronutrients (protein, carbohydrates, and fats), fiber, and added sugars. Research suggests that individuals who regularly read nutrition labels tend to make healthier food choices and have better overall diet quality.

Case Study: Sarah's Path to Healthier Eating

Sarah, a 35-year-old marketing executive, struggled with weight management for years. After being diagnosed with prediabetes, she decided to revamp her diet and lifestyle. With guidance from a nutritionist, Sarah learned how to interpret nutrition labels and make wiser choices at the grocery store.

By prioritizing whole foods, lean proteins, and high-fiber options, Sarah successfully shed excess weight and improved her blood sugar levels. She attributes her achievements to the changes she implemented in her grocery shopping routine, emphasizing the importance of planning ahead and adhering to a shopping list.

Tips for Successful Grocery Shopping on a Diet:

Make a List: Before heading to the store, assess your pantry and fridge, and compile a detailed shopping list. This will help you remain focused and resist impulse buys.

Shop the Perimeter: The outer aisles of the supermarket typically feature fresh produce, lean proteins, and dairy products. Prioritize nutrient-dense foods from these sections for a healthier shopping experience.

Read Labels Carefully: Take note of portion sizes and ingredients listed on nutrition labels. Avoid products high in added sugars, saturated fats, and sodium.

Choose Whole Foods: Opt for whole grains, fruits, vegetables, and lean proteins over processed and packaged foods. These options are typically lower in calories and richer in nutrients.

Conclusion:

Grocery shopping while on a diet is a skill that can be refined with practice and knowledge. By comprehending nutrition labels, planning ahead, and making mindful choices, you can transform your shopping trip into a journey towards improved health. Remember, the decisions you make at the grocery store can have a lasting impact on your overall well-being.

Chapter 20: The Power of Journaling While on a Diet

Introduction :
Embarking on a journey towards a healthier lifestyle often involves making changes to our diet. While the prospect of transforming our eating habits can be daunting, one powerful tool that can greatly aid in this process is journaling. In this chapter, we will explore the benefits of journaling while on a diet, backed by data, numbers, insights, and case studies that highlight its effectiveness .

The Impact of Journaling on Dietary Habits:
Research has shown that keeping a food journal can significantly enhance the success of a diet plan. According to a study published in the American Journal of Preventive Medicine, individuals who tracked their food intake through journaling lost twice as much weight as those who did not. This striking statistic underscores the importance of mindful eating and the role that journaling can play in promoting awareness of our dietary habits.

Numbers Don't Lie:
In a survey conducted by the National Weight Control Registry, which tracks individuals who have successfully lost weight and maintained their weight loss, 75% of participants reported that they regularly kept a food journal. These findings highlight the correlation between journaling and successful weight management. By documenting what we eat, we are better able to identify patterns, triggers, and areas for improvement in our diet.

Insights from Experts:
Nutritionists and dietitians often recommend journaling as a valuable tool for clients seeking to adopt healthier eating habits. By recording meals, snacks, and beverages consumed throughout the day, individuals can gain insight into their overall caloric intake, nutrient balance, and areas where adjustments can be made. This process of self-monitoring can empower individuals to make informed choices and stay accountable to their dietary goals.

Case Studies:
To illustrate the real-world impact of journaling while on a diet, let's consider the case of Sarah, a 35-year-old professional looking to lose weight and improve her health. Sarah began keeping a food journal, noting down everything she ate and drank each day. Over the course of four weeks, Sarah noticed a pattern of late-night snacking and excessive sugar consumption . Armed with this newfound awareness, she made targeted changes to her eating habits, such as swapping out sugary snacks for healthier options and practicing portion control . As a result, Sarah not only lost weight but also experienced increased energy levels and improved overall well-being.

Conclusion :
In conclusion, the practice of journaling while on a diet can be a game-changer in achieving and maintaining a healthy lifestyle . By documenting our food choices, we become more mindful of what we eat, identify areas for improvement, and stay on track towards our goals. The data, numbers, insights, and case studies presented in this chapter serve as a testament to the transformative power of journaling in the realm of dietary habits . So pick up a pen, grab a notebook, and start journaling your way to a healthier you.

Chapter 21: The Power of Probiotics : Enhancing Your Diet for Optimal Health

Introduction :
In the world of health and wellness , probiotics have gained widespread recognition for their numerous benefits . From improving gut health to boosting immunity , these live bacteria and yeasts offer a plethora of advantages for overall well-being. In this chapter, we will explore the role of probiotics in enhancing your diet while on a weight loss journey. By incorporating probiotics into your daily routine , you can optimize your digestive health , support your weight loss goals , and improve your overall quality of life.

The Impact of Probiotics on Weight Loss:
Numerous studies have shown that the balance of gut bacteria plays a crucial role in weight management . A healthy gut microbiome can help regulate metabolism , reduce inflammation , and improve nutrient absorption —all of which are key factors in achieving and maintaining a healthy weight . In fact, a study published in the International Journal of Food Sciences and Nutrition found that participants who consumed probiotics experienced significant reductions in body weight and body mass index compared to those who did not .

Furthermore , probiotics have been shown to reduce cravings for unhealthy foods and promote feelings of fullness , making it easier to stick to a balanced diet and avoid overeating . By supporting a healthy gut microbiome , probiotics can help create an environment that is conducive to weight loss and overall well-being .

Real-Life Success Stories :
To illustrate the impact of probiotics on weight loss, let's look at a case study of Sarah, a 35-year-old woman who struggled with obesity for years. After incorporating probiotic -rich foods such as yogurt , kimchi , and kefir into her diet , Sarah noticed significant improvements in her digestion and energy levels. Over time , she also experienced gradual weight loss and found it easier to maintain a healthy lifestyle . By prioritizing her gut health through probiotics , Sarah was able to achieve her weight loss goals and improve her overall quality of life.

Probiotics and Digestive Health :
In addition to their role in weight management , probiotics are also essential for maintaining a healthy digestive system . These beneficial bacteria help break down food , absorb nutrients , and prevent digestive issues such as bloating , gas, and constipation . By promoting a diverse and balanced gut microbiome , probiotics can improve gut motility and support overall digestive function .

According to a study published in the Journal of Clinical Gastroenterology , participants who consumed probiotics experienced significant improvements in symptoms of irritable bowel syndrome (IBS), including abdominal pain and bloating . These findings highlight the importance of probiotics in managing digestive disorders and promoting gut health .

Choosing the Right Probiotic Supplements :
When it comes to selecting probiotic supplements , it's essential to choose high-quality products that contain a diverse range of beneficial bacteria strains . Look for supplements that are backed by scientific research and have a high colony -forming unit (CFU) count to ensure optimal

efficacy . Additionally , consider consulting with a healthcare professional or nutritionist to determine the best probiotic strain for your specific health needs and goals .

Conclusion :
In conclusion , probiotics offer a myriad of benefits for individuals looking to enhance their diet while on a weight loss journey . By incorporating probiotic -rich foods and supplements into your daily routine , you can support your gut health , improve digestion , and facilitate weight loss . With the right approach and guidance , probiotics can be a valuable tool in achieving your health and wellness goals . Embrace the power of probiotics and transform your diet for optimal health and vitality .

journal writing : where plots thicken and hearts lighten !

journal writing : where plots thicken and hearts lighten !

journal writing : where plots thicken and hearts lighten !

journal writing : where plots thicken and hearts lighten !

journal writing : where plots thicken and hearts lighten !

journal writing : where plots thicken and hearts lighten !

journal writing : where plots thicken and hearts lighten !

journal writing : where plots thicken and hearts lighten !

journal writing : where plots thicken and hearts lighten !

journal writing : where plots thicken and hearts lighten !

journal writing : where plots thicken and hearts lighten !

journal writing : where plots thicken and hearts lighten !

journal writing : where plots thicken and hearts lighten !

journal writing : where plots thicken and hearts lighten !

journal writing : where plots thicken and hearts lighten !

journal writing : where plots thicken and hearts lighten !

journal writing : where plots thicken and hearts lighten !

journal writing : where plots thicken and hearts lighten !

journal writing : where plots thicken and hearts lighten !

journal writing : where plots thicken and hearts lighten !

journal writing : where plots thicken and hearts lighten !

journal writing : where plots thicken and hearts lighten !

journal writing : where plots thicken and hearts lighten !

journal writing : where plots thicken and hearts lighten !

journal writing : where plots thicken and hearts lighten !

journal writing : where plots thicken and hearts lighten !

journal writing : where plots thicken and hearts lighten !

journal writing : where plots thicken and hearts lighten !

journal writing : where plots thicken and hearts lighten !

journal writing : where plots thicken and hearts lighten !

journal writing : where plots thicken and hearts lighten !

journal writing : where plots thicken and hearts lighten !

journal writing : where plots thicken and hearts lighten !

journal writing : where plots thicken and hearts lighten !

journal writing : where plots thicken and hearts lighten !

journal writing : where plots thicken and hearts lighten !

journal writing : where plots thicken and hearts lighten !

journal writing : where plots thicken and hearts lighten !

journal writing : where plots thicken and hearts lighten !

journal writing : where plots thicken and hearts lighten !